Pink Tears

Patricia Newsome

Copyright © 2023 Patricia Newsome

All rights reserved. No part of this book may be reproduced or transmitted in any form or by any means, electronic or mechanical, including photocopying and recording, or by any information storage and retrieval system, without permission in writing from the publisher.

Published By: Publishing Advantage Group
www.PublishingAdvantageGroup.com

Table of Contents

Introduction 4
Chapter 1: The Beginning 9
Chapter 2: Times of Adversary 14
Chapter 3: Moving Forward 21
Chapter 4: New Life, New Friends, Same Story 24
Chapter 5: Back To Where We Started First 29
Chapter 6: Time for a Change 36
Chapter 7: In a Dark Place 42
Chapter 8: Again, God showed me what to do… 46
Chapter 9: Matthew 18:19 49
Chapter 10: Life Changing 51
Chapter 11: The Diagnosis 56
Chapter 12: Had to Quit to Fight 60
Chapter 13: God is Real 68
Chapter 14: It's a Blessing and a Curse 71
Chapter 15: Full Circle 82

Acknowledgements

First and foremost, I would like to thank God for allowing me to prosper through this Journey. I am amazed by and constantly reminded of his grace and mercy, without him there would be no miracles.

Next, to my two beautiful daughters, Tabria and Tabijah, as well as both of my God Children Shay and John, thank you for encouraging me through my ups and downs which gave me strength and more perseverance. I love you all! Thanks for never giving up on me.

Thank you to my parents, my siblings and Family for being supportive of me. I gracefully show my appreciation for all your prayers and the love you've continued to display through my experience. I sincerely appreciate the calls and text as well as stepping in during my time of need.

I express my gratitude to Tyquan Harper and my friends for their constant words of encouragement and support.

I am grateful to Abecka and express my gratitude for you opening your home to me when I had nowhere to go and the healthy meals you prepared for you and my children. Most of all thanks for the laughter we shared when I wasn't feeling well.

Joy and Lashunna, I thank God for giving me the opportunity to meet you both. Remember you are braver than you believe and stronger than you seem. It's your life and your story, keep your faith and always keep God first. Much love!

R.I.P to my Children's father Tabios and the memories that we created, shared, and learned from. We miss you every day. (Nuthnbutluv)

Mr. Kelly Cole and Publishing Advantage Group my appreciation goes out to your team for being patient with me through our writing and editing process. Now we are here. Thank you and Blessings!

Last but certainly not least, I would like to give a huge shout out and thank you to Jemile Weeks, Director of Wefam United, for allowing me to volunteer for your organization to help underserved youth and families in our community. You give everyone who works alongside you an opportunity to grow and discover their purpose. You're a tremendous leader and have inspired me to seek what I love and do what I enjoy which will lead me into my divine purpose.

Introduction

I often reflect on my life and all that happened to me. I sometimes reflect as a spectator and acknowledge that most people would not have survived all I have been through. Loss, extreme grief, abuse, and survived a fatal illness. Every decision I've made and every situation I was in puzzled me when they were happening. I did not understand why God was allowing me to experience life like this. Now I realize that every second of those experiences shaped me into who I am today. Those things didn't happen to me, they happened for me. They happened so I could share this story with you. This story is a story about faith, perseverance, obedience, and trusting in God. I want people going through similar experiences that I went through to know that God has a plan, and to trust that plan. Had I not given God full control of my life, I would not be alive today. My prayer is that this book, and my story, is encouraging to you all.

CHAPTER 1

The Beginning

I was born and raised in Lakeland, Florida, a small town between the cities of Tampa and Orlando. While Lakeland is often called, "American's Town" because of its extraordinary beauty consisting of 19th-century-styled homes, streets lined with beautiful oak trees, and thousands of acres of delicious orange trees, grapefruit trees, and sugar canes. While the beauty was heavenly—Lakeland was one of the most violent places for African Americans to live.

Both from other parts of the deep south, my parents supplied a rich and nurturing home atmosphere that was filled with love, respect, and integrity. Contrary to the general narrative of African American families, where the father is absent from the home and the mother is struggling with several children, that was not my story nor the state of most of my relatives and friends. I lived in a wonderful home of a hard-working father and a spiritually grounded mother. My dad was the typical strong, honorable, and hardworking southern man. He labored long hours at *Empire Construction* company. When he came home, my mother and siblings remained quiet while catering to our father's needs. Very seldom did my dad raise his voice, but when he did, look out.

I remember listening to the late-great James Brown, whom we called, the "Godfather of Soul," that was singing a song entitled, "Papa Don't Take No Mess." One of the lyrics describes dad 100%, "Papa didn't raise a whole lot of fuss, but when we did wrong, Papa beat the hell out of us." That was my dad. Mom was a strong Black wife and mother. She made sure that we cleaned the house and did our chores. She instructed us on how to fix traditional African American meals that included okra, mustard greens, steamed dumplings, catfish, and the kind of southern fried chicken that Colonel Sanders would beg to eat. While dad was the quiet storm that ruled by imagery, mom was a hands-on disciplinarian, she gave us insight into early life lessons like the importance of being on time, having manners and making sure we studied our school and religious lessons and attended Sunday School and church every Sunday. We had numerous restrictions like not being able to leave the premises of our house, never being allowed to do sleepovers at our friends' houses or to go trick-or-treating during Halloween or getting involved with recreational or extra-curricular sports. The major point to remember is that I had a nuclear family with five siblings. We never went hungry, homeless, or naked. My father did not beat my mother, nor abuse his children. We were not wealthy, but rather, the typical Black family in Lakeland. Going to church on Sunday in Black America, especially in Florida before the 1990s, was an event. It was a time to socialize with friends, gossip, and of course, thank God for his blessings. We treated attending like an outing, wearing our finest "church clothes."

Pink Tears

The traditional African American church, unlike today's megachurches, was filled with residents who took the church and its lessons seriously. We attended a church called Macedonia *Primitive Baptist Church* and typically arrived at 8:30 am for Sunday School followed by the 11:00 am service. My brother and sisters all had their special classes, while my parents went to adult classes. After Sunday School, the children and teenagers congregated to chat before the church service started. The black church is the greatest of traditions of our people. The structure, style, and soulfulness of the nature of black spirituality is something that we as a culture often appreciate. For example, to the left of the preacher's podium sat the trustees, stewards, and deacons. To the right, were the missionaries in their white dresses. In the front rows were the mothers of the church and the preacher's wife, with her big hat and loud-colored, tight dress. Now, depending on the Sunday—one of the choirs would sit behind the preacher's chair. I occasionally sang with the young people's choir. Our services would last sometimes up to two hours. The music, pageantry, sermons, and the dancing to the "Holy Spirit" is the experience of the black family and black church, forming one bond of spirituality. Oftentimes the excitement of the church service would follow us home, we would sing make beats by hitting the back of the seat with our hands and clap. When dad was feeling the spirit, he would bring out his guitar once we got home trying to model the rhythms of the famed Mighty Clouds of Joy, dad would play such tunes as, "*We Come This Far by Faith,*" and "*I've Been in the Storm Too Long.*" While our family was rooted in the black church spirituality, our faith was often tested as a unit. For instance, I once handled my father's guitar and broke a string he told us to never touch his instrument again. However, on one special evening, that fine guitar looked like it wanted me to touch it, -and I did. I guess I was feeling like my father's favorites, BB King, or Lita Ford—I plucked a few strings, thinking that it was sounding good, and did it a few more times. Well, you can guess what happened next, a string broke. When my dad found his string broken—he became as hot as a firecracker. Being the first child that he saw standing by his baby—the guitar, he asked me if I broke the string? In a frightened, lying tone, I responded no to the question. He asked my other siblings and, of course, they said no too, but *they* were telling the truth. We all got our butts beat that night. The guitar for my father was his tool for relaxation and family time. Instead of watching television, listening to the radio, or scanning the internet as contemporary families of today often do, dad would gather the family together to sing. Sometimes, the songs would be gospel, other times we would sway and sing the blues. Being a real child of the 1980s and 1990s I loved the music of LL Cool J, Public Enemy, and Queen Latifah. Like any other child I followed the styles and sounds of urban modern society, even though I lived in the hinterlands of Lakeland. The beginning is the foundation of what type of person you are going to be, and it plays a major part in your adulthood. It is responsible for making you grow into the woman you are supposed to be. Our parents, childhood experiences, and unfortunate events will influence the direction our life will go. Do your beginnings define your future? I would soon find out.

Train up a child in the way he should go and when he is old, he will not depart from it.
Prov. 22:6

CHAPTER 2

Times of Adversary

My best friend in school was Anita. She was a well-focused girl who always wanted to join the military. Throughout our teenage years, we spoke for hours about what branch of service we were joining and what our future would look like when we got into our twenties. What made her my best friend and deepened our friendship was how she helped me get through the death of my younger sister. It was during my sixth-grade year. In the early morning, I was awakened by a commotion from my parents' bedroom. The sounds of screams, crying, and loud footsteps disrupted the normal peace patterns of our small home. I, along with my brother and sisters, looked perplexed, not knowing what took place and what we should do. My aunt, Ann—was in my parents' room, while my cousins were sitting in the living room with fear on their faces. They were just as bewildered as my siblings, and I were. Aunt Ann was instructing us what to do and where to go but we were still confused.

I could hear my mom on the phone with the 911 dispatcher yelling, "Please hurry!" Frozen and polarized, we stood still while listening to my Aunt Ann pray in my parents' bedroom. My Aunt, just like us, was deeply religious. She was a "holy roller," as we said. That is, she received the holy ghost, spoke in tongues, did the holy dance in church, and prayed over people with spiritual oil. So, when she was praying in our home, we knew something had happened. Through the sequences of, "Dear Jesus!" "Lord help us!," and chants from her, I heard an ambulance racing through the streets towards our home. Within seconds of hearing the sirens, paramedics rushed through our home towards my parents' room. When they came out, they carried my baby sister Annlisha on a stretcher to the ambulance. Annlisha was a beautiful girl, joyful, and full of life and laughter. Thus, seeing her motionless body being carried away by strangers to the hospital was odd. My siblings and I asked silently, what had happened? Did she fall? Was she sick? Or even worse, did someone hurt her? I fell into shock. Not knowing what happened, I lost touch with parts of reality.

I remember riding in a car to the hospital, when we arrived our father stood in the waiting room Aunt Ann gathered my siblings, cousins, and me into a circle to hold hands and pray while my parents were with the doctors. About an hour later my parents came back to us and told us that Annlisha was gone and didn't make it. She was only eleven months old! Eleven months. She didn't even get to live one full year in this world. We were all shocked and confused. We didn't immediately comprehend what they meant by *"gone"*. That was my first experience with death. We drove home in complete silence. It was a *Twilight Zone* moment. Just two years ago, I finally mustered up the courage to ask my mom what happened, and she explained that Annlisha died from a genetic chromosome condition called *Edwards Syndrome*, also known as Trisomy 18. This illness caused her to have a heart defect. My mom added to my shock when she told me Annlisha was diagnosed at birth. Only my parents knew. My siblings and I had no idea. She didn't look sick to me. My parents were very private, even with their children. Sometimes I wish they would have at least shared that with us. I may have been more prepared and my first experience with death may not have been so traumatizing. Or maybe they thought we were too young to understand.

Death is a strange event in life. It can either bring a family closer together or tear it apart. Annlisha's death brought our family closer together, but we still wanted answers. While we were at the hospital, we prayed for God's intervention. We wailed for his healing powers that are expressed and illustrated in the New Testament. We asked God, *why Annlisha?* What did she do? But my sister died regardless of our cries to God. It tested the faith of our family and our beliefs. After the death and incredibly sad funeral, our home had the feel of a corpse, cold and lifeless. After some healing, our family grew closer together and we started taking family trips once a month. The trips were a nice distraction from the constant thoughts and questions about Annlisha. My parents were trying to bring the joy back. It helped, especially with us kids but I noticed the change in their relationship. Very few interchanges between my parents. Sometimes there was only dead silence between them. No more light flirtations, quick kisses they thought we didn't see, or sweet glances I would catch them throwing towards each other. It was a tough time for everyone in the house. The attempted words of comfort from my Aunt Ann, "Annlisha went to be with the Lord.", did not heal my wounds of hurt, rather, it made me sad, angry, and confused every time she said it. I simply could only ask, *Why God? Why Annlisha?* For a while after Annlisha's death, I read the Bible every day looking for answers. I thought about the times we shared and what she would be like if she had lived. I simply faded away into a dark depression over my baby sister's death, silently. I never spoke up because I was mature enough to know that my parents had been through enough and I didn't want to add my overwhelming sadness to their plates. I prayed and cried, cried, and prayed. Eventually, a vision came to me that my sister had become God's new angel. My friend, Anita was the only person I was able to talk to about my feeling with at first, but after my vision from God, I was able to finally start healing, after I was even able to go to my parents and ask them questions about death and the afterlife. We were all finally healing.

Now, while I was raised in a strict home that featured God as the center of our lives and discipline, I attended public Lake Gibson High School, as opposed to a Christian school. As a student, I always took my classes seriously. God gave me visions at an early age of me doing remarkable things with my life. I wasn't sure if my greatness would be in the U.S. Army (since I had thought about joining), academia, vocational, or business training, but I believed that I would obtain a phenomenal future. I was not extremely popular. I was cute and smart—but nothing out of the ordinary. I knew that some of my teachers thought of me as a student with potential, because of my studies and level of focus. During my freshman year of high school, I met Roy a senior. He was the typical cool, handsome, rough, bad guy. He was the dude you didn't need but you like. Roy was completely different from me. His family life was unsettled and dysfunctional. They didn't know God. He was often suspended from school for fighting and went to jail for criminal activities early on in his adult life, but —Roy made me feel special like an older woman. So, who cared if my folks disapproved of my relationship with him, my mind was already made up. My friend, Anita, said that Roy was *trouble* she said he was too old and had no future. Like many young women, I broke the girl code and negated my friendship with Anita, for my love of Roy.

By age fifteen, Roy was my world. He was a hit to most teenage girls. It never jelled with me that Roy was explicitly attracted to teenage girls. As I got older, I began to realize that it is easy to manipulate girls who are as my mom would say 'too fast for their britches.' At that stage in life my friendship with Anita and my parents were all secondary to Roy. In my mind he loved me as well as he loved his family. and ultimately my father wanted to kill Roy, and then me. My father could not believe how rebellious I had become and how this jerk was with his 'baby girl'. I remember thinking, 'What's the big deal? I was 15 and Roy was 19!" He was fearless. In Lakeland everyone had a hunting rifle and no one was afraid to use them, especially daddies. It is a small town where people love to shoot everything from rabbits to deer It is the culture. Thus, shooting a man dating a younger female is fair game. My father probably wanted to kill Roy, just to keep him away from me but he didn't have to worry about my Christian father shooting him My father's tactic was to try to keep me busy with more chores and school activities. I believe he thought keeping me busy would: 1. Leave me little to no time to see 'Rusty Roy' as my dad called him, and

2. Make Roy see he was too old and find another girlfriend. I was willing to do or say anything to keep Roy in my life. I did the unthinkable and told my very first lie to my parents. I had my bright idea all planned out. I was going to tell my dad, 'Daddy, I am pregnant.' Although my father and mother would be extremely hurt and angry about me being "pregnant," I had to believe that they were too much of Christians to kill the father of their grandchild…at least I hoped so. It seemed logical and understandable to my 15-year-old brain. So, for weeks I faked morning sickness, loss of periods, and pregnancy mood swings. The justification—save Roy from jail. I never imagined the trump move by my mother—taking me to our family doctor. The physician, sternly and quietly, informed my mother that I was not pregnant. The test was negative, which I knew already. Roy and I had never had intercourse. My parents were furious. My Dad stressed that he was disappointed in me, and that Roy was not a good guy. To my dad, Roy was a coward, which was why he could never meet with him face-to-face, man-to- 'man.' Roy ended up robbing a store and was sentenced to 5 years in prison. When he was released, he attempted to rekindle our relationship. He hoped my 15-year-old brain hadn't developed, I guess. Thank God I had matured by then and was able to tell him no. I moved on with my life and had more sense and higher standards. My point is that my father was right had I ended up with Roy, or having his child, my life would have turned out horribly different. Roy free, I was preparing to move to Orlando to start a new life full of new opportunities.

Do not be deceived: Evil company corrupts good habits.
1 Corinthians 15:33

CHAPTER 3

Moving Forward

In June of 1994, I graduated from Lake Gibson Senior High School. It was a beautiful and exciting moment in my life. My Mom, siblings, friends, and classmates were all there with excitement, joy, celebration, and optimism about what was to come. Graduation meant change it was the opportunity to leave my family, friends, and town in the pursuit and exploration of a new world. A world of new dreams, education, and career. It was my liberation; the only sad part of this event was the fact that my father did not attend the graduation services. I believe that the drama and trauma that I took my dad through were extremely hurtful to him. Stupid, young, and immature I did not realize how much I had insulted and hurt my father. I didn't even have the integrity, honor, and respect to apologize to my father as the man, and leader of our household. To this very day, I wished that someone would have instructed me to do so—without regard for my arrogance or hurt. Now I have the courage and integrity to tell him, so here it goes, "Daddy, I am sorry for the pain that I caused you and the family. I was young and dumb, now that I am older, I understand the world you were trying to protect me from. You were only looking out for my best interest. Because of your selflessness and love, I became strong and confident with what I can do with my opportunities and dreams. No matter where I go in life, or what I do, there is always a part of you in my heart. Thank you for loving me forever. I love you.

Shortly after graduation my cousin Nikki and I decided to move to Orlando. The city was as beautiful as the residents. Vastly different from Lakeland, Orlando was a world-class community in central Florida and the home of over one million people. Moving to Orlando meant meeting a diversity of people and exploring attractions like Disney World and Universal Studios. The great educational activities of educational institutions such as the *University of Central Florida*, and *Florida A&M University Law School*, a variety of clubs from hip hop to Jazz, underground, caused Nikki and I to be thrilled. My parents understood my move they offered me simple, but powerful advice— "Be careful, always remember God, and center on your upbringing." Lakeland to Orlando is approximately 70 miles in distance. However, it is a world apart. Everything from employment, education, entertainment, population, and people.

Nikki and I shared a small two-bedroom apartment with her cousin, Angie, from her dad's side of the family in a downtown neighborhood called Paramore. Paramore, often called *The Hood*, a term that I used, but didn't reflect the make-up of the community. It is a diverse community of African Americans, Puerto Ricans, Arabs, and Whites that reside at the economic lower end of society and struggle every day with low-paying jobs, inadequate housing, few city services, and street crime. One of the reasons the community has a reputation as a decaying society is because of city politics. Over 80% of the city's homeless population is forced to live in the Paramore area, while most of Orlando's bars, strip joints, and homeless shelters are in the neighborhood. Regardless of how people viewed the community—it was an exciting place and period in my life. In the area where I lived, it was common to hear conversations in Haitian Creole, Jamaican Patra, Spanish, or African American Ebonics. In other words, Orlando was hip, cool, and soulful. We fantasize about getting jobs, and meeting new and exciting people, while also building our contacts and learning our way throughout the new area. This whole turnaround was God-directed. During my activities and newfound freedom, God was molding me into something wonderful and great. I recognized the hand of God in my life at that moment and I paused to thank him for extending the grace I did not deserve. I put my past behind me and focused on my future life. This was only the beginning of the story of my imperfect adulthood.

For we know that if our earthly house of this tabernacle were dissolved, we have a building of God, a house not made with hands, eternal in the heavens.
2 Corinthians 5:1

CHAPTER 4

New Life, New Friends, Same Story

I adapted fast to my new life. It did not take long for me to find a job. I was hired at Popeye's restaurant on the heart of the Paramore strip. One of my parents' characteristics that embodies my DNA was the quest to be independent. Thus, getting a job illustrated the pillars of freedom and stability. So, there I was with my new life new job, and new friends. I was naïve enough to believe life could not get any better than this. I loved making my own decisions and feeling free for the first time. The thought and the feeling of being liberated from all restraints was an emotional high. Plus, working at Popeyes was a plus. The type of characters that entered through the front doors piqued our interest. For example, one minute would be church folks coming to order food, and then the next minute it could be the rude belligerent customers. Eventually, Nikki was hired at Popeyes too, and boy we had fun. We made new friends that would alter my life. There were a group of young men and women who were between the ages of 19 to 25 who came into the job frequently. They were "street," but cool. The way they would come into the restaurant joking around like it was their second home made them look like a fun crowd to hang with. They were very reflective of their city and went by the name of the *DTO* which stood for Downtown Orlando. The DTOs seemed to like me and Nikki, so we eventually started hanging out with them. Many of the guys were older than us these are the people we bonded with because they were acceptive, protective, and positive. Most of the time we just hung out, rapped, and sang, speaking about the ways of the world and black folks. The rap and sounds that we attempted to imitate came from the beats of Warren G, Snoop Dog, and Marshall Mathers-positive sounds, self-help, and freedom. Much different than the misogynistic lyrics of "gangsta rap." With a musical background myself, it was not long I, too, was dropping beats. I always had fun and funny moments hanging out with the DTO Crew. We all had a lot in common. They gave me the nickname "Peewee" because I was the smallest one in the group. At first, I did not like the nickname, however, the endearing term represented a special place for me. I was the little one from a small country town, who was reared in a sheltered environment. Therefore, all the guys treated me like a little sister. They looked out for me they protected and encouraged me to do the right thing. While I liked the DTO, another group came along that stole my interest—they called themselves, the *Long Street Posse Crew*.

They were "street smart" and tough. Different than the DTO, who spent their time with musical beats. The Long Street Posse Crew were slick hustlers who often bent and occasionally broke the law for self-gratification. They were also very protective of me but in a different way.

Pink Tears

The Long Street Posse Crew was known on the streets as "hustlers." If you bothered one of them—you had an "ass-kicking" coming from all of them. No one dared to disrespect me because I was now a part of the crew. —Simply put —they ruled their territory. A lot of shootouts took place and illegal drug deals. They lived an extremely dangerous lifestyle in the middle of the hood. Knowing all of this and now being a part of it, I still hung with them. Why? Because they were "cool," and I liked them.

I began dating one of the members by the name of Torrence. Our romance sparked after I jokingly took his beeper one day and he told me to hang onto it so that he could beep me later. He was handsome, medium build, had never been in trouble with the law, book smart, and was loved by everyone. While being with this new crew, I felt like I was in one of the "hood" movies I used to watch on TV. I was living the real-life *Boyz n The Hood*. It felt surreal that I was welcomed into their lifestyle—it was exciting! When they entered my life, things got interesting I never imagined myself being in these kinds of dangerous situations like, "drive-by" shootings on both sides—being around the shooter and being the victim. I was now living a wild, but exciting life. For example, sometimes at house and block parties as alcohol, drugs, and weed were consumed —emotions, attitudes, and fights broke out. I'm talking, fists flying, and sometimes guns being drawn. However, I was never afraid but rather excited which added to my quest to join the U.S. Army.

Several months later, Nikki, and I went to a recruiter in Orlando to enlist. The Recruiter spoke about military benefits, opportunities, and travel. We immediately did the paperwork and scheduled the required physical. During my physical examination, I found out that I was pregnant. This time it was true! This news crushed me as well as my dreams of traveling and hopes of fighting for my country. At least I thought so at the time. I knew I needed a plan B. No, not as exciting as the US military, but durable. The tough part at this stage was telling Nikki that I was not joining her in the quest to become an American soldier. We moved to Orlando together, now we are separating. When I told her—we both were upset. We cried knowing the possibility that we may never see each other again. At the end of the day, Nikki had to follow her heart. She could not worry about me. I too had a destiny now and I had to follow my heart too. Motherhood.

After the cry with Nikki—I had to tell my boyfriend, Torrence. My mind was racing with the most important question-will he be accepting of our child? He put all my worries at ease.

Torrence was excited, proud, and elated. His "homeboys" threw us a serious party to celebrate the pregnancy. The party was live—music, dancing, food, and libation. I was overjoyed but I still had to focus on plan B for my life. Every choice we make in life determines our future. Think of life like a garden and planting seeds in our garden as choices. The seeds you plant are what will grow. Don't expect to grow apples if you planted lemons.

But this I say, He which soweth sparingly shall reap also sparingly; and he which soweth bountifully shall reap also bountifully.
2 Corinthians 9:6

Pink Tears

CHAPTER 5

Back To Where We Started First

I enrolled at *Valencia Community College* to become a Medical Assistant. Believing in the traditional family of two parents raising a child, I moved in with my man—Torrence. But the dreams of a single-family home with a white picket fence were dashed. Our home was a "trap house." It was filled with illegal drugs that ranged from crack to marijuana. It was visited and used by drug pushers, crackheads, and prostitutes. Our security was not ADT, but rather the 9MM, Uzi, and .45 and caliber *semiautomatic. Most people who occupied our space were from the streets. As my parents often stated, "Once you've made your bed, you must lie in it." Indeed, it was a hard bed.

One of Terrence's friends, Daquan moved in with us and got into some serious trouble. He would stay in during the day and run around gingerly at night. One of the nights that he ventured out, he was spotted by one of Orlando's finest—the Orlando Police Department. When he saw the police, he instinctively ran. Not asking any questions, the police ran after him. During the pursuit, OPD released a round of ammunition into Daquan's back. He died instantly. OPD justified the murder by stating they mistook Daquan's beeper for a firearm. He died just a few blocks away from our home. We were all devastated and traumatized by his death. It became clear to me then that death had no limitations for who it took. First, my sister died as a baby, then Daquan was in his twenties. Both gone too soon. So naturally, at this point, I was stuck between a rock and a hard place. I was pregnant and going home to my parents was not an option. During this drama, I never lost faith in God and apparently, God did not depart from me. His mighty wings were covering and protecting me. If not, I would have gone completely insane.

Despite everything I was going through, I continued to focus on my education, employment, and my unborn child. Eventually I told my parents about my pregnancy. My parents were disappointed, knowing this was not the example they set for me, but they remained loving and supportive. Although my living surroundings were less than admirable Torrence and I were doing great. We were happy and expressed deep and sincere love for each other as we awaited our bundle of joy. About five months into my pregnancy, I found that I was giving birth to a girl. I was so excited, and she was all I could think about—purchasing cute pink outfits, creating a lovely baby room, and her first baptism. However, the most important thing that escaped me was a name. What would I call my baby? One of Torrence's friends, "E" suggested the name Tabria, "Tabria." It was a unique name, and the meaning engulfed my thoughts of my baby girl. Tabria means, beautiful and goddess, gift of God. Indeed, such a name would require the responsibility of both me and my daughter to live up to such a unique name. A few weeks later as I was leaving the house, still in bliss daydreaming of my unborn daughter, my peace was interrupted by a cadre of cars embarking on my location at a high rate of speed. Although it momentarily shook me—I thought nothing of the vehicles until I turned a corner and headed to our house. What I saw was frightening! Unmarked and marked police cars had our house surrounded as armed members of the Orlando Police department SWAT team rushed into the house. Emotionally, I wanted to rush in and help my man, but physically I was frozen—scared stiff I could not move. I waited nervously outside. After more than an hour Torrence, our friends, and customers came walking out bound by handcuffs. It seemed so surreal to me to see everyone being placed into a police van. They all were arrested and charged with drug trafficking and distribution. Standing there with tears flowing down my face, I asked myself, ``What am I supposed to do now?" This was not a part of plan B, and I hadn't thought of a plan C. If I had waited five minutes before leaving the house, I would have gone to jail myself.

My heart raced with the thought of me almost going to prison, delivering my child as a convicted criminal, and then having my baby taken from me to be placed as a ward of the State. It was a heartbreaking thought. Uncontrollable sobbing, and in shock at what a bullet I just avoided, Torrence now in jail I ended up leaving the house and moving in with Torrence's Aunt Loretta. I felt so secure and welcome as she helped me get to and from work. She would even let me borrow her car to visit Torrence in jail. She even allowed me to cook my favorite soul food dishes like okra, collard greens, candied yams, and smothered pork loins. Everyone always enjoyed my cooking, and I would always credit Mrs. Loretta for my skills with that Shepherd's Pie. Mrs. Loretta, as I called her, was the coolest, sweetest, and most sincere person. Even though I was going through all these changes, my best friend, Anita, was still there for me and she would come to Orlando once a month, sometimes more, to visit me. I enjoyed her company and the time she allowed me to spend with Jon, my godson. He was growing up so fast. On one visit she told me that she was pregnant and that I would be a godmother again. I was overjoyed that she was having a daughter.

About three months had passed before Torrence and his associates were released from jail. However, the State had to drop charges due to a lack of evidence to prosecute. We all agreed that the police were so eager to arrest Torrence and his friends, that they made an assortment of mistakes, and it forced the state prosecutor to forfeit the arrest and charges. Sometimes technicalities are good. After his experience of being in jail for the first time, Torrence wanted to make sure he stayed out of trouble. He got a job in construction. After a few months of us living with Aunt Loretta, we both moved back into the trap house, yet again! We planned to save our money and move away from the madness around us. Nothing was going to stop Torrence and his "homies" from throwing a house party. Of course, they got "wasted". Here I was five days away from my initial due date when my water suddenly broke. I could not wake Torrence up because he passed out, due to drinking the night before. I got up to see if anyone else in the house was awake, but just as I figured, everyone had passed out from drunkenness. There was no phone in the house, so I had no way to call for help. The contractions kept coming back-to-back. I attempted to wake Torrence again, and again I was unsuccessful. I got dressed and left the house, and I walked over to the next street where Torrence's brother, Q, and mother, Mary lived. I asked Q if he could take me to the hospital because my water had broken. Of course, he wanted to know where his brother was. I avoided eye contact while telling them that Torrence was at home and passed out from drinking all night. The contractions were stronger than ever by the time Q dropped Mrs. Mary and me off at the hospital. I did not know being pregnant was going to be like this. After 45 minutes of waiting, the nurse took me right back to the delivery room. Minutes later Torrence arrived. As I got undressed and lay on the bed, the nurse proceeded to check on how far I was dilated. The contractions were getting worse. I began to cry, saying I could not take the pain any longer. The nurse finally shouted, "Oh my, you have dilated 9cm already and you are about to have your baby—like now." Another nurse yelled for the doctor to come in immediately and then the nurse told me, "Try not to push." My heart began racing, everything was happening so fast. With all that pressure below, I could not help but begin to push. One nurse was begging me to stop, but I pushed, nonetheless. Before long, the baby's head popped out while the nurse was still crying for the doctor to get there. Just as the body of the baby was completely out, the doctor arrived to literally catch the baby girl. The doctor said I was right on time, and he began to laugh. All the nurses laughed too, but I was in too much pain and did not find anything funny.

Pink Tears

Our baby girl started crying, which was a relief. The doctor placed my daughter on my chest. Giving birth to a new life was so precious and I was so excited. Torrence could not stop smiling. At that time, we decided to name our baby girl, Tabria. After a few days in the hospital, back to the trap house, we went with a brand-new-precious baby girl! All I wanted to do was move out of this place. I wanted to feel safe now that I had a new baby. As weeks went by I was still unable to go back to work. Torrence worked—but continued to drink and party with his "boys." It started to become annoying—I simply stayed in my bedroom while they smoked and drank all day.

One frantic-eye-opening morning, the unthinkable happened. I woke up to a rifle with a red laser pointed right in my eyes. *What the hell?* My whole life flashed in front of my eyes. I was not sure if I was being robbed, attacked in a revengeful act, or if it was a sick joke. But it was the Orlando Police again! With my daughter in one arm, the police shouted for me to put my hands up where they could see them. I was so scared, thinking if I made the wrong move my daughter and I could be shot. It was horrific. I followed the officer's command. Moving slowly with my daughter still in my arms we got out of bed. The officers took us to the living room and sat me on the sofa. I was still holding my daughter in my arms. What was surprising to me was that Tabria and I were the only ones in the house. I was wondering where everybody else was. I glanced out the window of the living room and Torrence and his friends were watching from across the street in their cars as I was about to go to jail. They avoided going back into the house because they knew drugs and weapons were in the house. Since the police had already raided the house there was not much that they could do but be patient and watch how I handled the situation. All I could think was, ``*Why me?*''

Things were not looking good. I thought jail was surely in my future and my innocent daughter would be in the state's foster care system. Living in a trap house with drugs and other criminal and immoral activities. The officers began to question me, and I genuinely did not know anything. An officer found some drugs and threatened that the state was going to take my daughter. He asked, where did the drugs come from? I answered, "I don't know.," which was true. I was grateful for not knowing. Now they were looking for more drugs, weapons, and even money. I sat quietly, praying. "Lord, please take me out of this situation. I am scared." After hours of searching and questioning, the officers released me while telling me to leave the house immediately. "Don't come back to this house." I followed their advice and left. With everything that was going on in my life, I never told my parents or siblings. I did not want to be criticized.

Sometimes we find ourselves going back to the situation that was never good for us from the beginning.
TN

CHAPTER 6

Time for a Change

There is an old saying, "God, protects children and fools." Well, I was not a child—just a darn fool. I was determined that I would never again place myself in the company of people who had a great chance of being arrested. Nonetheless, I was determined to find better accommodations and a house. So, Torrence, Tabria, and I moved in with Aunt Loretta once again. She remained sweet to me and was never judgmental. Of the many lessons Aunt Loretta taught me, the most important lesson of all was the importance of being "real" to myself first. Meaning, that I must have focus and direction to achieve the best in life and not let anyone deter me from my future. With that in mind—I set out to find a small apartment. After several months of living with Aunt Loretta, saving money, and becoming a better woman and mother I was ready to move out.

With the grace of God, hard work, and a little luck, I was approved to lease a two-bedroom apartment. It was just a few blocks away from the trap house, which worried me, but at least it was *my own* place. Things were falling in place. Home is where the heart is. My daughter—Tabria,

Torrence, and I, the center of my heart—finally had a place to call home. We painted and decorated the rooms, purchased new furniture, and made our nine-month-old's room perfect for her to enjoy. A few weeks later we purchased a car, things were going so well that it felt too good to be true. Sadly, after a hiatus from misery, hell reappeared. Torrence returned to his old ways again, drinking, partying all night, and hanging out with his old street buddies. The smell of alcohol and street life turned my stomach. I constantly reminded him that we were parents, and we must be mature enough to leave the "ways of the world." He would not listen, or he did not care. He continued to come home drunk, and wild, and started to become abusive. I hated that his actions would create an atmosphere of loud arguments, profanity, and violent physical explosion. No matter how much I disliked his behavior, I was hooked and stupid for this man. Is it true that "love is blind"? During fighting and loving, then loving and fighting, I found the energy to purchase a gun. I really cannot explain the full reasons for the drive to buy a firearm. But I purchased a small 22 semi-automatic that I could put in my purse. The weapon empowered me greatly. I felt safe, strong, and confident once the gun was mine not because I had the courage or the ability to shoot someone, but rather, because it was my protection. Someone had to protect the house when Torrence was out late at night. His behavior of running the streets had the potential of turning our small living quarters into a trap house. His actions were obvious, and his street activities attracted a lot of attention, especially from the cops.

One day I gathered the courage to confront Torrence about his behavior. I waited for him to come home from a night of drinking and partying in my mind—*this was it!* As I waited for Torrence, I looked out of the kitchen window to spot him walking across the field with his friends, E and Berg. Feeling empowered with the new gun that I carried in my purse, I placed it in my jacket pocket. I ran to meet them halfway. I went after Torrence with heat and loud words of profanity. Torrence, drunk as usual, responded by screaming, "Crazy bitch, I'll kick your ass." Boy, I was hot. E tried to make peace between Torrence and me but was unsuccessful. Torrence picked up a brick and threw it through the back window of our car. I snapped in an instant, I pulled my new 22 caliber gun on my Torrence. Crying, shouting and cussing I told Torrence that I would shoot him. *I will kill you*, were the thoughts in my mind. At that point, I did not care about my child, parents, hell not even about myself. My mind went blank. Everything from this point was moving in slow motion. It was like a movie—a deadly scene. I cocked the trigger back to fire, and I pushed the gun hard against the temple of Torrence's head. He was nervous and stood there in silence with his eyes closed. My hand was steady. I slowly squeezed the trigger. I was ready to hear a bang, and see blood explode from his cranium. Instead—a sick sound of "click." In a split second, Torrence snatched the gun and floored me with a single punch. It was a complete knock-out.

Once I recovered from being knocked out, I asked, "Where's my gun? E told me that he took it and would hold onto it until Torrence and I both calmed down and did not kill each other. I was still angry. I held visions of calling the police, but I could not. Not because I had a firearm, with no gun license. I threatened great physical harm intending to commit murder. The point is that I could have been placed in jail. Listen, do not ever purchase a gun without a firearm license and proper training on how to handle a firearm. I still think about how I almost threw my life away. I had to escape—leave this toxic relationship. So, to avoid any more arguments and violent scenes I decided to move out. Within an hour I packed Tabria and my things and moved in with some friends from the DTO crew. Torrence and I were finished. At this time, I hated him. I did not want my daughter to be around her father. To me—he was a bad influence, dangerous, and a terrible dad. After a few weeks of leaving, Torrence started calling me constantly trying to get back. I did not care. Nothing mattered—how much game he talked; I did not care about the sex my only concern was escaping to a better place the trail of events was pure hell. Thinking over the events of being on the verge of being a murderer or a victim of killing someone caused me to pause. It was only through God's grace that I survived. Strangely I had to thank God for allowing Torrence to knock me out. Before y'all start tripping, I am not saying it's okay for men to hit women. I'm saying it was God's intervention that allowed me to escape the dead place in the quest for a better setting for myself and our daughter. I was determined never to allow anger to dictate my actions again. Therefore, I got rid of the gun was too easy to use such a violent weapon to handle concerns and issues among friends, family members, and the general community. I decided that day—I was going to recommit myself back to the spiritual foundation that my parents had drilled into me as a youngster. I went into the bathroom to wash my face and wipe those tears away. It was time for me to show my gratitude toward the heavenly father. I prayed constantly, thanking God for saving Torrence and my life.

Reviewing the tenants of Christianity, especially the concept of forgiveness—I called Torrence and apologized for the events that took place between us. I had to follow God's law and humble myself for my part in this drama. It was not about Torrence but me. Don't get me wrong, I was still done with him yes, I forgave him but my days of being a fool were over, so I thought. Carnal love is a terrible temptation. One thing about street brothers-they are smooth. Lust crept back in and after 4 months of being separated I gave him another chance. He also used the "I miss our baby girl" line on me. The next thing I knew —I had packed my bags and moved in with him again. Secretly, I wished that someone like my parents would have intervened to stop me, but they truly had no idea of what I was going through. Even though I thought that I knew what was good for me—I was simply responding to my heart and my physical needs.

Once I got back home, things *were* better. Torrence did not hang out with his friends as much and we started to do things as a family. We went for walks, had picnics at Lake Eola—downtown Orlando, we even spoke about the Bible and spirituality. Finally, I thought that we had made a turn for the better. Thus, with a new heart, and a clear mind I increased my hours at my job to save money so that we could purchase our first home. Within 6 months after getting back together I saved enough for a deposit on our new home. Excitement was in the air. Everything was working out so well. The house, which was in a better section of Orlando, was far away from the physical drama that Torrence and I had gone through. Life was good and getting better and I continued with my education.

A time for change means we must grow from our old ways. Back to the "garden," I mentioned earlier. I was planting good seeds because I was determined to grow, I had to remove myself from the bad soil-let go of the old dirt to prepare for the new I felt deep in my heart and soul that I deserved better.

The fruit of the righteous is a tree of life, and he that winneth souls is wise.
Proverbs 11:30

CHAPTER 7

In a Dark Place

Now, back to Torrence. Things were going so well that I ignored the fact that Torrence was "slipping back to darkness." Perhaps, being jealous of me working long hours or just feeling the urge to "be the man," he started to become more controlling physically and mentally. That is, using aggressive and degrading language, bossing me around, and insulting me in front of friends. Not to mention he accused me of cheating if I refused sex. As if that was not bad enough—he was drinking heavily again, especially on the weekends. These days were terrible. He would drink with his buddies, and come home for sex, and arguments. It was as toxic as an environment could get. It got to the point that when Torrence came home, I could tell when he was drunk or not by the way he would slam the front door. It was obvious that I was weak for Torrence. I knew that he would not change, but I believed, like so many women, that I had a special power, some sort of juju that would reform my man. I lied to myself and anyone who would listen to me say that this man would change I prayed and asked God why he did not make me strong. My exact questions to God were, "God, what did I do to deserve this brut of a man?" "What happened to me?" My father and mother are God-fearing people. I was raised in a strict God-fearing home. My dad never disrespected my mother. "God, how did I get into this fix?" "Why would I, you allow a man to treat me in such a vile and evil way?" Sometimes the actions of a man who is full of anger and violence encourage a woman to question themselves. They lose themselves and their focus on life. Even though I had an excellent job, a beautiful daughter, and a new house, I hated myself.

    I fell into a dark place. An area that was in the deepest, darkest corner of hell. I used to wonder how and why people committed suicide. I often wondered how a celebrity who had it all; money, houses, cars, popularity, and fashion would kill themselves. Now, I knew—the feeling of loneliness, feeling hopeless and not seeing another way out of the situation. On a day of feeling lost, sad, and spiritually and physically worthless, I picked up a gun and placed it on my head. I wanted death, but at the same time, I was too fearful of pulling the trigger and leaving my daughter behind. Looking back at that situation I realized that God was allowing me to change my life once again. It was his voice, his conscious that told me to put the gun down. With tears running down my face, at that very moment, I knew my life was not over. I was at a place in my life with no one to talk to that wouldn't judge me and my situation. I am not a child of the world, but rather, God's child. He made me realize that failure does not mean that I had failed in life. It means a step of evolutionary spiritual and mental change. The change is quick, tough, and drastic. For instance—I tried reaching out to associates and friends from the DTO crew, but they left me alone. They hated Torrence, some even wanted to beat his "ass." They had become tired of telling me to leave him, only for me to end up staying. Thus, they decided it was on me.

My excuse to them concerning my lack of strength in leaving Torrence was my daughter. That is, I did not want my daughter to live without her father. My plan was to remain passively silent. The fact was, I was afraid of him after his nights of drinking and still very much in love with him. I decided that when he came home drunk, rude, rough, and hostile, I would remain silent. Hoping and praying that he would not physically assault me. However, it was not working. That is the same with Torrence, he was not going to change his behavior unless forced to. Knowing this, I was still so foolish. Would you believe that I got pregnant again? *How could this be?* I was not ready for another baby. Heck no. I had a job, bills, and an unsettled dysfunctional relationship. *Damn, another baby with this man?* After a while, I felt better about the living growth in my belly, our baby. When Torrence realized that we were having another child, it seemed to get better—again. That is streaks of kindness, concern, and love. There were fewer arguments, and we took time to talk about the family's budget since I would be taking time off from my job.

In July 1999, my healthy 6-pound baby girl, Dyshea was born. We were overjoyed to have the baby. We all fell in love with the addition to our family. Amid this drama, I received one of the worst phone calls of my life. My best friend, Anita, had died. Wow, that was a blow. My high school classmate, the same "sista" who was there for me since day one. A woman so full of life and destiny—dead? How? *Why God?* I had become tired of asking this question. I had been asking for it since I was a child when my baby sister died. *Why do you allow good people to die, while giving evil people full sway into the lives of others? Why are you taking them while they're so young?* I cried a bucket of tears. I asked—aloud, "Who is going to take care of her two beautiful children—Jon and Shae?" I just could not believe that she passed away. Feeling blue and emotionally unbalanced because of her death, I attempted to talk to Torrence about it. Boy, it was the wrong move. He responded with no empathy or concern. I was expecting him to comfort me like Anita did when my baby sister died. At the very least, I expected him to comfort me as my man. I should have known better. Now, after being in our new home, fussing, fighting, and enduring his lies and cheating ways for eleven years—I was through with this man. Tired, fed-up—Torrence had to go. I was serious this time. The flame finally went out. It was time to let go. I had to remember that God is the head of my life. I had to start loving it and putting myself first. A part of me knew he needed me. It was easy to take care of everyone else, but I didn't take care of myself. Taking care of yourself is not to be confused with holding down your own. Yeah, I could pay my bills, keep a job, and all the essentials of being an adult, but I had no clue how to realize when I needed to be taking care of myself. It would be years before I learned this.

But the fruit of the Spirit is love, joy, peace, longsuffering, gentleness, goodness, faith.

Galatians 5:22

CHAPTER 8

Again, God showed me what to do…

This time I took God's advice and told Torrence to move out. Of course—he was reluctant to leave, but at the end of the day, he didn't have a choice. It was my house, in my name and my name only. Once he left, I vowed never to talk to him again. I did not care that he was the father of my children. All I knew was that he had caused too much pain, hardship, and frustration and I was determined to end the madness. Finally, I was liberated. Of course, it was difficult physically being alone—without Torrence, without a man. But like Mary J. Blige once said, "I can do bad all by myself." Now all my energy was placed into my children. All that they wanted and needed was stability, a loving environment, and peace. With Torrence, that simply was not possible due to all the drunkenness. The children forced me to focus on real goals and objectives. I was pushed by them I could not let them down. Resiliency had become my friend and the essence of my moral character. Often when friends saw me, they remarked about my new attitude and strength. I just responded with, "It's perseverance baby!" Shortly after Torrence was out of my life, I finished school and earned my medical assistant certification. I then enrolled at an institution to earn my degree in Nursing shortly thereafter. Unfortunately, the continued cost became a financial burden. At that stage in my life, with Torrence gone, everything was on me. Yes, it was tough childcare, education, housing, and food, all came from one source—me. However, I must not ignore the role of God—his hand was guiding me. I once heard a reverend say, "Jesus never spoke in a church and that he never pastored a church." The point is that I did not go to church while all of this was going on. Yet, God blessed me. My children were happy, healthy, and excellent students, so things were good. My attitude became, "who needed church and church people." Heck, the ultimate blessing was a year later meeting a tall, dark handsome man named, "Corey."

I met Corey at the mall. This brother held the mall door open for me with a big, lovely smile. Immediately, there was a spark in a conversation, and we exchanged phone numbers. For weeks we spoke on the phone about serious and silly things before making plans for our first date. Then later we dated seriously for five months before I introduced him to my daughters. In the one year of dating, we moved in together. Our relationship was great. Attentive to my daughters and myself, Cory was a hardworking, respectful, and loved God. Corey referred to me as his "queen," and surely, he was my "king." Every day with him was a vacation. We never argued, used profanity, or criticized each other in front of the children and the public. Yes, we had some serious disagreements, but we always remained civil. Time flew by because we were having so much fun. Despite this great atmosphere (soil) and five years of living together—he wanted to have kids and I did not want to, so we decided to end our relationship. My experience with Torrence was traumatizing and I did not want to have another child out of wedlock. To be honest, I was still trying to find my inner me. We would still be friends, but without benefits. Thus, I was single again. My girls are now in middle and high school. Tabria, the oldest daughter, graduated from high school with honors and started college at FAMU in Tallahassee, Florida. She honored me in front of a large cheering crowd with the words, "Job well done, Mom." My baby girl Dyshea was doing great in school. She took all honors classes and became the captain of her middle school cheerleading team. Before I knew it, I was teaching Dyshea to drive. I don't know where the time went but I knew we were happy, and my girls were going to do great things in life. The next chapter in my life came with Abby. While working at dialysis I met a young lady who was interesting, exciting, and humble. Immediately, we struck up a conversation and eventually became good friends. She became a benefactor if anyone needed anything, Abby was there. She would ultimately be my angel. I bring her up to once again show that God never left me alone. As alone as I felt at times now that I am reflecting I realize that God always sent me angels, Anita, Aunt Loretta, and Abby.

To everything, there is a season and a time to every purpose under the heaven. **Ecclesiastes 3:1**

CHAPTER 9
Matthew 18:19

In late November 2013, my favorite cousin, Walt went to the hospital because he was having breathing problems. When I heard that Walt had been taken to the hospital, I rushed to Lakeland to see him. When I arrived, the nurse informed us that Walt was in a coma. It was a strange scene. Doctors nor nurses could tell us the reason Walt had fallen into a coma. All we could do was pray and wait for a miracle. My aunt asked her church for special prayers, while I continued spiritual salutations to God as I consistently read Matthew 18:19: *"I say unto you, that if two of you shall agree on earth as touching anything that they shall ask, it shall be done for them of my Father which is in heaven."* I repeated the scripture several times, day and night. Indeed, I was looking for intervention from the forces of heaven. As I waited and looked to God to use his mighty power to save Walt—our sweet Walter passed away two months later, having never regained consciousness.

Although God had saved me in the past from hostile relationships, dangerous environments, drugs, criminal activities, and suicide, I began to think of God as being ineffective after Walt's death. My walk with God became weak. So was my understanding of God's ways, he always answers prayers, but we think the answers should match our desires. Persons of faith know that if we hold fast to our beliefs and trust in the Lord everything will work out as it is supposed to, and God will get the glory. I knew all this intellectually, but my heart was so broken that all I could feel, see or hear was pain. I knew I no longer wanted to walk that faith walk anymore.

I realized that "walking by faith and not by sight" is much easier said than done. My faith was replaced with pain, hurt, and anger. *Dear God, where are you when I need you?* I would have given anything to hear Walt laugh, and joke again. I was hurt and in disbelief. It was hard to come to terms with the fact that he had passed away. My outlook on life changed and my views on God changed. Why take my troubles and burdens to God? He does not answer prayers. I know exactly where to go if I need answers- Straight to a damn liquor bottle. Yep, vodka and Hennessy were my communions. *God, for real? Please, he was an imaginary being with no real power. However, if by chance he existed. He does not care about me.* Those were my feelings, my thoughts at that time. Like James Dean said—" the good die young, while the bad live long lives." So, I began living in the world and started drinking and clubbing as I pleased. Why live a righteous life and pray? I would've rather go drinking and doing what I wanted to do because God do not answer prayers. As if the pain of losing my closest cousin Walt was not enough to handle, my life was about to change in ways I had never dreamed of.

"Jesus immediately reached out his hand and took hold of him, saying to him, "O you of little faith, why did you doubt?" **Matthew 14:31**

CHAPTER 10

Life Changing

(The Phone Call)

On December 3, 2014 one year later and ironically Walt's birthday I did a self-examination on my breast. I discovered a lump the size of a grape on my left breast. It got my attention. Why? Because it was not there a month ago. Now note while I doubted and lost my faith in good God, I did have enough sense to regularly check myself for breast lumps.

You see it's funny that while I was busy cursing God now, I might have breast cancer. I prayed like a child praying for a shiny new bike for Christmas. I apologized to God. I wondered if God was testing me, or maybe was punishing me for my sins. If he was punishing me for my sins. *Am I being prepared for something greater?* I did not know all I knew was that I could not sleep, eat, or do much else.

When I finally fell asleep, I had the mother of all dreams or perhaps a vision. God spoke to me saying that I was going to experience the biggest and toughest fight of my life. If I follow God's directives, I would be placed on the top of the mountain top. My testimony would go worldwide. Yes, I am being tested by God for my terrible ways. Sometimes we believe that

God does not respond to our evil ways. Yes he is all-forgiving, but that does not mean that God does not occasionally punish us for our transgressions. I woke up exhausted, but with a different feeling. I still grieved for Walt—but I had to now understand the workings of God. Not only did I gain a better understanding of the nature of God, but I felt his presence and power. For instance—I felt an immensely powerful force within my body as well as externally. His forces sent me to my knees as I cried and begged for God's forgiveness. At that moment I comprehended what pastors and missionaries had said throughout the years, "God is patient, but he is a jealous God and that we should put nothing before him." Yes, that wonderful and great force called God—could have allowed me to die, become a drug addict, a whore, a thief—but he saved me. A person who should not have been given a second chance. I can say with clarity that God not one of his angels, not a prophet, but the man himself had sought me out and visited me. When I got up from my knees I felt like a new woman. I will not lie and say that I became perfect right away, but I came to believe that I will be a servant of God. That was the best one-hour prayer that I ever experienced. I understand that nothing happens without the will of God.

    When I woke up the next day, the thought of me having breast cancer was overwhelming and the worst feeling ever. My thoughts were *will I beat this or die from this disease?* I was scared. I showered, dressed—skipped breakfast, and went directly to Dr. Carr, who is my primary care doctor. Without an appointment, I waited for over two hours. In strange—while being nervous about the lump I was also extremely calm. Eventually, the

Pink Tears

doctor examined me. Immediately I was ordered to get a sonogram and a battery of other tests. Once completed—the doctor and associated medical professionals ordered a biopsy to be done on the lump the next day. Immediately, my mind was triggered, *this must be bad. A biopsy?* Well, the doctor explained to me that an incision will be made on my breast to remove a sample of the tissue for testing. Although they stated that the area would be numbed, I expected pain. The procedure went on without any problems. For the next few days, I was a bundle of nervous energy. Yes, I prayed and felt comforted by God, but my earthly nature ignited various thoughts of gloom and darkness. To fight the darkness, I read selected scriptures from the Gospel. I reflected on God's visitation with me, and I knew that I was not alone. I understood that God, the Father, and the Holy Ghost stood with me as I would prepare for the greatest challenge of my life if my test results came back positive.

Now, don't get it twisted—was I afraid? Yes. Fearful? No. I was now in the bosom of God. The difficult part was telling my family that there is a chance that I may have cancer I did not want to hear the general old thing: "Don't worry." "Everything will be fine." Sometimes people with the best motives can say things that make you feel worse. So, I tabled the discussion for another time. Truth is, I did not want to be in an atmosphere that was filled with "cancer" talk I wanted to have fun and relax. On my visit to my parent's home, I did not inform anyone of my challenges with the biopsy. After leaving my parent's home, Dyshea and I decided to take a road trip the next morning to see my grandparents in Alabama. Driving to Alabama from Florida is a beautiful feeling. Passing and driving through geographical

Pink Tears

differences, one cannot help but notice the beauty of lush green fields, the rolling hills, and the deep appeal of southern culture and etiquette. The drive was spiritually healing. Dyshea, enjoyed the road trip—it was the bonding that we needed. One of the things about a long road trip is that you have time to think and talk. It is a refreshing experience-almost spiritual cleansing. Along the way Tabria called several times to check on us and to make small talk but when I was quiet, I thought about the chances of me having breast cancer. One of the interesting things about this disease is that it forces you to be humble. That is, we typically think about day-to-day activities, materialism, and simplistic arguments and chatter. It registered that I could be dead in a few months. What would my children do? Will their father step up to guide them in the right direction? Everything was racing through my mind. Should I take a once-in-a-lifetime trip with my children? So many questions. So many thoughts. I wished this were a bad dream, but I knew it was not. That was my reality at the time. Nothing but death, cancer, and my children filled my thoughts any time I was not engaging in a conversation with someone else. In many respects, I wanted to tell my grandparents what was going on. My grandparents are great. They listen, they support, and they encourage. I decided not to say anything when I arrived at their home. I only showed love, hugs, and tears. My grandma and grandpa were wonderful. Living in the back hills of the south and living off the wholesome foods of God—my grandmother prepared outstanding meals. Fish and grits, bacon and eggs, greens, cornbread, chitlins, and rice, are foundational foods. Meals in Black southern culture poured out of her kitchen. Listen, when you eat *real* fried okra and smothered chicken you can never go back to Kentucky Fried Chicken, Popeyes, or Maryland Fried Chicken. Southern Black food is simply the best. My grandparents' southern cooking was incredibly good for my soul.

After enjoying the wonders of southern cuisine—I still labored on the disease that might be growing inside of me. I was happy and sad. I was polarized, in and out of consciousness. Busy thinking about, "what-ifs." Still, I remained "cool, calm, and collective. "As I was sitting down in the kitchen speaking to my grandma, I received a telephone call from the doctor. It has been nine days since they took a biopsy. The physician stated that I need to make an appointment for this week. My heart was beating fast. I knew this was not good, and I knew I had to continue to enjoy my time with my grandparents before I headed back home the very next morning. Time passed so fast that it was time to head back home to reality.

For I will restore health unto thee, and I will heal thee of thy wounds, saith the LORD; because they called thee an Outcast, [saying], This [is] Zion, whom no man seeketh after.
Jeremiah 30:17

CHAPTER 11

The Diagnosis

The next day I was at my physician's office. The longest wait that I ever had for a doctor's appointment and so much anxiety. When the nurse told me to enter the examination room and wait for the doctor, and that I was almost done I felt that I was going crazy. Dr. Carr walked in with a look that could kill a brick. In a monotone he said, "I am sorry, but you have Stage III breast cancer." *How? Why? What? Are you sure? I want a second opinion.* Were all my thoughts that I could not formulate into sentences. Devastated is not the word that I experienced it was a feeling that turned my stomach inside out. I was angry no, hostile at the news. Now I had a new date to remember besides my birthdate—December 12th. The date when I was told I had "invasive ductal carcinoma stage III cancer." Now I had to seriously think about planning for my children after my death. But first, how will I tell my children? Family? Friends? Darn God—why are you always putting me in an unpleasant situation? I asked for forgiveness, yet I had stage III cancer. This suck.

The physician knew my frustration, but I had questions. *How soon am I going to die? What can be done to save my life? What is next?* Immediately, the physician referred me to an oncologist. He stressed that I make an appointment and start my chemo treatments.

As I was leaving the office with a pile of informative material and my test results the receptionist with a sad smile whispered, "You will be okay, let God handle this." Yes, if God had my back. If God was handling this, I would not have cancer. That is what I thought but was immediately redirected as I remembered that the father said that I was going to have the biggest fight of my life. Jesus said in the book of Matthew, *"Truly I tell you, if you have faith as small as a mustard seed, you can say to this mountain, move from here to there and it will move. Nothing will be impossible."* Yes—I was still mad. I did not fully understand why I was being singled out. I asked God once again for forgiveness and told him, "Your will shall be done. After a good cry in my car and trying to rationalize God's motives and even suggesting that He made a mistake. I settled down and remembered what my aunt told me after the death of my sister "God does not make mistakes."

I was not sure what to do or where to go. Instinctively, I drove to my sister Keke house—she was headed to her mailbox I got out of the car and stood frozen. Seeing the distress on my face she asked what was wrong and I burst into tears sobbing that I had stage III cancer. She hugged me and cried too. She told me, "You're going to be okay." Then asked, "When are you going to tell your children?" I did not answer. I was not ready. Tabria is in College and Dyshea is in the ninth grade and having a great year as a captain on the cheerleading team. I did not want to interfere with my children's activities. Like Mike Tyson stated, "Everyone has a plan until they get hit." My mind was all over the place, I didn't want to stay at my sister's, but I also was not ready to go home.

Once home I was sitting in a chair in my bedroom brainstorming. Dyshea walked in. In a split second I started crying. My daughter asked, "what's wrong?" I cried, whaled, hollered, and then screamed out that I have "cancer." In my bedroom she became an acting mother at that point. Calmly she asked did Tabria know. Then she said with a warm smile and hug "Mom, you are going to be fine. You are the strongest person I know, and I will be with you every step of the way." In response to her sister not knowing, we had Tabria on the phone within minutes. I broke the news to my first born and with an instant pause that seemed like an eternity, she initially said nothing. Then I heard crying and she said she was coming home to be with me, but I asked her not to. I told her "Finish what you started and Complete the semester." Truthfully, I wanted both of my girls with me. Regardless of my illness, I had to look out for their best interest. It was not about me even though I had breast cancer. My next position was to figure out what came next.

Words are powerful. We must be careful what we say when we speak, we must go start speaking positive in our lives because God can heal anything we just have to pray, exercise faith and grace. I had to prepare my mind for the fight of my life. I knew that I was not just fighting for myself, but I was also fighting for the people who depend on me. For me, I wanted to fight for my girls.

He sent his word, and healed them, and delivered [them] from their destruction.

Psalms 107:20

CHAPTER 12

Had to Quit to Fight

We often take the beauty of the world for granted. The beauty of the moon, stars, sun and rain. The joy and freshness, When I was told of my diagnosis, I began to see the beauty in the world. I did not know if I would be seeing the beauty of God's creation much longer. But surely—I had to direct my life and focus on my children and daily activities. Once more I turned to God. I am glad that he is merciful and forgiving. You talk about backsliding, as you can see—I was the queen of backsliding. But I prayed for strength and courage, because I had heard so many stories of the disease taking over the lives of the victims as well as their family unit. I found out I had family members that had or died from breast cancer. I wonder if I would have known, maybe I could've done something to prevent it from happening to me. The older generation in the African American culture always kept secrets. I think information on health should be told to our younger generation so they can be aware of their chances of any health risk. This generational cycle stops now, starting with my children. They will have information on my diagnosis. Meanwhile I cried for many days and nights, but I knew that I had to stop. I realized that through the grace of God, I would not let cancer control my life. I made up my mind that "I exist, I live, so I will win," I will beat this.

I went to my first oncologist visit. Dr. Flow and I discussed the details of my diagnosis and the type of treatments I would need during my fight to survive. The type of breast cancer I had is called Ductal Carcinoma, which is the presence of abnormal milk duct in the breast and is considered the earliest form of breast cancer. The cancer had also spread in my lymph nodes under my armpit which are called micrometastases. According to a study conducted by the *American Cancer Society* in 2022, about 1.9 million women will be diagnosed and about 609,360 women will die from breast cancer in the United States. My oncologist was highly informative. I was still in disbelief and wanted a second opinion Dr Flow offered insight and recommendations. My doctor concluded that I had an aggressive form of cancer. She deliberated and concluded that once I start treatment I should stop working, especially since I worked with sick patients. I thought about my immune system and infections and reluctantly took her advice. So, right after my doctor's appointment I went to my place of employment to meet with my supervisor I informed her of my diagnosis. In a snap she responded, "What about your job?" I wanted to drop her with a left hook. This is when it fully kicked in that I had to learn to care for myself. My job to whom I gave so much of my loyalty and devotion only cared about staffing not that I could potentially die. I rolled my eyes, gave her that sister stare and said in hood fashion," Do what you have to do." It was painfully clear—most people don't care about your troubles, hardship, or pain. We live in a cold-blooded society. I knew who I could emotionally depend on called my parents, my children, and scores of family members and friends. These were the people I knew cared about me and would not take it personally that I was finally caring for myself. My attitude was set now. I am not ready to die.

In a few days I returned to my physician for a "port placement" examination. This procedure determines the placement of chemotherapy injections in the body. I did not like the term chemo, but I had to live. This will be my first surgery ever, the thought of sleeping while someone or a group is probing your body is strange. It is a bit freaky and somewhat violating. One week later it was time for my surgery. My children and Torrence met me for the procedure and stayed with me. They quickly became my pillars in this episode. As they waited outside the room for me to undress, wipe my whole body with these sterile wipes from head to my legs as the nurse instructed, and prepare for surgery afterwards my family was allowed to be with me until the nurse called me to a special area for pre-surgery. As I was taken into a designated area for surgery, I remember praying nonstop. The anesthesiologist came in to explain what he was preparing to do for me. I tried to focus on what he was saying but I didn't realize he was injecting the medication while talking about doing it. I was out in an instant. The procedure took an hour to place the tubing in my upper right chest area. My daughters and Torrence were there waiting for me to wake up after the surgery was complete. I was feeling so dizzy that it took me a minute to gather myself together. A few hours after my procedure I was released from the hospital with pain medication. Afterward, Torrence helped me to Tabria's car, and we went our separate ways for the day. I was exhausted but grateful the surgery went well without any complications. It had become official Chemo was now part of my life.

On the 31st of December 2014 I started my first Chemotherapy treatment. There wasn't going to be any dancing through the New Year, no viewing fireworks, or drinking wine. Instead for me a treatment room, a nurse, a scale for preparation, and a chair to wait my turn for Chemo. Wow! This is it. With both of my daughters and Cory by my side I will be fine.

My name was called, I read the details, and shortly after a needle was placed in my new chemo port. *Are you kidding me?* This needle hurts. I screamed out in pain and briefly lost composure. However, when I looked around the room to see if anyone had noticed my emotional outbreak—no one seemed to care. Everyone was in their zone dealing with their own set of problems. *What? Am I the only one scared? Should I be showing my emotions? Am I a weak woman?* In a flash of those questions came an answer I cannot beat myself up the medicine is going to do that. Sitting in a chair with multiple medicines running through my veins and next to me was an IV pole with nine bags hanging from it was bazaar and weird. It felt as if I was in some strange experiment. Nonetheless, during those four hours I went to the restroom several times with the IV pole and the iv lines still attached to my chest. Eventually, on the fifth and last time I returned to my seat and fell asleep. When I woke up and read the orders that I needed to follow a transformation developed. I knew there was more I needed to know other than what I was given to me to read so google became my best friend. I studied the type of cancer I had, the survival rate, and the chances of it spreading. In addition to my Google research, I read a litany of materials about cancer, treatment, diet, and exercise programs. However, the most significant was learning about cancer and sugar. I found out that sugar was the fuel for cancer. That is cancer cannot live without sugar in your body. What is interesting and a paradox is that as time passed the nurses at the Cancer Center gave out candy and soft drinks. From this moment I had to change my mindset and diet. Therefore, at home sugar was out! No candy, soft drinks, cake, or anything that contained sugar. Immediately home was a sugar-free zone. Along with no sugar I said goodbye to meat. No hamburgers, steak, hotdogs, ham, and pork ribs. I began to purchase foods high in antioxidants, drank lots of water containing alkaline with PH 9.5 with Electrolytes and at this point I found myself shopping at an all-natural foods store. This is where I found my organic turmeric, herbs, and elderberry roots. I started a regiment of terrible-tasting herbal teas like Essiac and Green tea. I did not care about the taste; it was about living. See turmeric and elderberry can be found in a powder or root form. It has several health benefits including fighting cancer. With my essiac tea, I had to boil it and drink 8 oz 3 times a day and plenty of water. I would prepare meals like breakfast carrots, avocado, blueberries, or plain oatmeal with no sugar. Dinner was sometimes egg plants, baked chicken, and broccoli. I would eat 2 meals and throughout the day I ate fruit that was beneficial for fighting against cancer. I started making beet juice blended with ginger and carrots. I studied what foods were high in antioxidants that help fight against cancer and other diseases. To name a few; blueberries, blackberries, avocado, beets, papaya, red apples, soursop, red grapes, spinach, kale, collard greens, and ginger. Each of these I did every week in rotation. I stopped drinking alcohol and intake of all dairy products. Anything that contains sugar or fried foods was a no for me. It was hard to let go of that 2 piece-spicy chicken and a biscuit from Popeyes, but I had to stay consistent with my eating. I also started exercising two times a week or whenever I had the strength. I also studied foods that increase your risk of breast cancer which were fast foods, fried foods, processed meat and other processed foods that are refined in carbs. Along with all the effects of cancer I now have a list of new medications.

Of course, I had to follow the medication orders from my doctor. One was a product called Neupogen, which helps produce more white blood cells after chemotherapy destroys some of them. This medicine is usually given 24 hours after every chemo treatment. With every new procedure I had to undergo, I found myself praying that everything would be fine. As I sat in a designated chair and watched the nurse remove a small vial from the refrigerator. She injected the Neupogen in my right arm, which gave me a burning sensation. The first night after receiving the Neupogen injection what I experienced was brutal. I was in so much pain. My arm felt like it was placed in a meat grinder. It was so bad that I started to have a headache. I went to bed trying to sleep off the pain but after a few hours of sleeping I awoke in a cold sweat. My pajamas and linens were drenched in water. I got out of bed and attempted to change my pajamas and linens. As I got out of bed and started moving a sharp pain ignited in my back, the pain was unbearable. Immediately, I lost my breath. What *the heck is going on?* It was strange and a mystery to me. I decided to take a cool shower thinking that it would dull the pain. It did not work. I was up-all-night crying—the pain was bad enough for me to go to the hospital. Dyshea knocked on my room door to check on me because she could hear me crying. She wanted to help in some way but we both knew there was nothing she could do. I told her pretending the pain had subsides "The only thing you can do is pray for me baby." Dyshae responded with, "I am always praying for you, mom." We both bowed down on our knees and prayed. Dear God, we *know that You are the one that heals and supplies all our needs. You are the one that delivers us and sets us free when in trouble, I run to You. Set me free because You are a good God like You say in Your word, please Take my pain away Amen.* Finally, after hours of being up I fell asleep. As the morning sun began to rise and shine brightly in my eyes, I realized I had made it through the night and was beginning a brand-new day. I remembered a passage in the Holy Bible that says, "We may weep for a night, but joy will come in the morning." When I got out of bed, I was pain-free. I just looked up and gave the Man above my praise. I was not embarrassed to shout and sing praises to the Lord for stopping my pain. He had answered my prayers. Since I was feeling better my daughters and I decided to go wig shopping. I knew before long; I would be losing my hair. Of course, I thought about all the beautiful bald African models. But at this stage I did not dare to wear a "baldy." After visiting several stores, we found a "rocking" wig. It was perfect. It looked natural and it was just lovely. I remember seeing older church mothers wear wigs and never thought I would be wearing one at the age of 39. It has become a part of my life now.

Pink Tears

Better is the end of a thing than the beginning thereof: and the patient in spirit is better than the proud in spirit.
Ecclesiastes 7:8-14

CHAPTER 13

God is Real

My cousin Carra had invited me to visit her church. I had not attended a church service in a very long time. I have been praying and asking God for assistance and forgiveness I was not a member of any denomination or congregation. For a long time, this was intentional. I felt it had nothing to do with my relationship with God I was following my own path and not God's. This time I was willingly and eagerly doing it in God's way. The "Mothers" and missionaries of Black Christian communities call it "the negative self-accusing spirit." While I suffered from this spiritual affliction when the deacons started praying and the choir began singing, I could not stop myself from praising God. My discomfort turned to a feeling that I belonged and that I was home.

The Pastor entered the pulpit area and the choir continued to sing an enormously powerful song that touched my soul. The Pastor began to preach his powerful sermon which spiritually moved the church. Then at the end of service the Pastor addressed the congregation and in a surprising twist he called my name and instructed me to come to the altar. I asked myself: *Is he kidding me? This pastor does not know me.* I was reluctant and a bit embarrassed. I had never attended this church. I do not know the people. The bigger question: *Why is he calling my name?*

Reluctantly, I got up out of my seat and walked up to the altar, it seemed like the longest walk in my life. Once at the altar the Pastor told the believers "I want to pray for the healing of this young lady." I wanted the prayer, but I was scared I did not know what to expect again I had never been to the venue before. How did he know me? Was it prophesy? I did not know.

Everything was so new as the Minister, the deacons, missionaries, mothers, and the entire church all joined in for congregational prayer. The pastor's prayer statements were becoming more intense with each breath. I started to sweat and became unbearably hot. A strange and powerful entity entered my body. It was possessed by the Holy Ghost. I'm not sure why, but my theory is that maybe spirits were fighting for control over my body, all of this was taking place while I was in a spiritual trance and state.

When the possession stopped, I am sure now that God was purging that sickness of cancer out of me the power of God is tremendous. I am testifying that spirits exist good and bad I tested God; I disobeyed him and lived an ungodly way. I only called upon him when I needed his love and salvation God the Spirit showed me that he was in control He is strong, I am the weak one. Right after the prayer, I ran to the restroom to vomit. The vomit came out a yellowish color and as I was experiencing these feelings and thoughts a lady in the restroom comforted me and gave me some water to drink, I was thirsty and tired. Carra soon came into the restroom to check on me. She too confirmed what had just happened the holy spirit was moving through this place. This honestly frightened me, and

I wanted to go it was an experience that I never expected. The lady in the bathroom stated before I left: "It's the devil trying to intervene on what the Lord is trying to do for you." Even though I was being purged of the evil of Satan, I must admit that I respected the power of the devil. Not in an effective way, but in a way that you respect a hurricane, snow blizzard, and earthquake. All activities are great, powerful, and potentially destructive.

I wanted to get out of that church fast, quick, and in a hurry. While I was walking to the main door to leave. I ran into the Pastor. The pastor invited me back to the night service. He said, "Come back to our night service because I have more for you. God has revealed much more about you to me, and I want to share it. Please come back." I nodded my head and continued out of the front door. I knew I was not planning to go back because I was scared and confused. The power of God is great, but also frightening. In retrospect, I should have gone back to give the devil a "black eye," as church mothers say.

After leaving church I headed back to Abby's house where I was living at the time. I told Abby about my experience, and she was in shock saying really are you going back later I said heck no. Abby was there for me and lifted my spirit when I got into my moments of sadness or not feeling well. She was God sent; she never asked anything of me, but to get some rest and take care of my health.

And they were all filled with the Holy Ghost, and began to speak with other tongues, as the Spirit gave them utterance.
Acts 2:4

CHAPTER 14

It's a Blessing and a Curse

Whether I was terrified by my church experience or not, something miraculous happened that I know was nothing but the power of God. Before I went to church, I had a large lump on my left breast. A few days after visiting the church, I had a scheduled examination with Dr. Flow upon examining my breast. In amazement and confusion, the doctor asked me what happened to the lump. She was puzzled and I was floored by the question. The look on her face illustrated extreme confusion. She knew that she examined me and that the lump we both felt, was now missing. Then she explained that it was "impossible for the lump to shrink so fast in such a short time." Her confidence was so broken that she called in her associate to review the previous x-rays that showed a cancerous lump. Instinctively, I thought of the pastor at Carra's church. It must have been the prayers, the Holy Ghost, and the exorcising of the demons that came out of me in a white-yellowish vomit. It was evil. The physician was talking to me, but I could not hear or understand what she was saying. My mind was on the church. The feeling of being hot, dizzy, weak, and losing consciousness. I am trying to understand what happened at that church. Now, I reflected on what the minister stated, "Come back there is a blessing waiting for you." I should have—but I didn't.

The physician, apparently not a person of faith, maintained that my chemotherapy must continue. During this conversation, she said that I must consult a plastic surgeon. Dr. Flow referred me to Dr. Lewis, a plastic surgeon. I was disappointed and I wanted it all to be over just like that. I now wanted to leave. I just vomited out demons, the lump has disappeared, and you're telling me I must continue treatment? I am on the way to getting closer to God. I contended that God would heal me and destroy the cancer that occupied my body. After visiting the doctor and leaving with more questions than answers, I walked over to start my second four-hour chemo treatment. Torrence stopped by to sit with me, but two hours into my treatment, I started feeling horrible. I was warned that chemo was an invasion of the body and had many negative side effects. But since my first treatment was not too bad, I assumed that all of them would be ok. Once again, I was wrong! More chemo was building up in my system and it was targeting cancerous tissue and good tissue as well. All I wanted to do was sleep the sickness away. After my treatment, Torrence had to drive me home. I was dizzy and drained. Meanwhile, I found the inner strength to let Torrence know how I felt about him after all these years of being with him. I told him I hated how he treated me, and took me for granted, but strangely, in the middle of what I thought would be a long rant about everything I hated about him, I found myself say that I forgave you. It was evident that God had found me. I was lost, and now I am found. I was now on a mission that was directed by God. Torrence apologized and stated he never thought I had that much hatred towards him. He said, "I guess that's why you never responded to my texts or calls." With a smile, he added, "Well, since you have forgiven me, you should give me another chance." My respond was simple and forward — "Don't push it." I was glad he apologized and admitted he was a failure in our relationship. He seemed to have matured and now understands the meaning of commitment and true love. I forgave him, but I will never forget the treatment and the hard times he took me through. I know you probably think when you forgive you are supposed to forget. We all are human, and we know you will never forget what someone has done to you. Nevertheless, during my cancer journey and afterwards Torrence and I became good friends once again.

    I arrived home. Showered the bad chemo smell off me I called it the smell of "death." For the remainder of the day, I did not have an appetite. It was a tough time. The effects of cancer and my treatments were now starting to show. Dr. Flow provided me with two different types of prescriptions; Temazepam to help me sleep, and an antidepressant med called Zoloft. There was no way I was going to take those medications just to have more health problems, so I didn't. Maybe I *was* depressed. I didn't want to admit to it. I just had to leave everything in God's hands. Let me tell you, having breast cancer was painful daily. The cancerous breast had consistent burning pain. It was like the cancer was burning everything on the inside of my body and there was nothing I could do to stop it. There were several issues I dealt with on many occasions.

    Many may not know that chemo can affect your memory. I remember driving home one day in an area well to me. As I was sitting at the traffic light, it dawned on me that I had no idea where I was heading or where I was. I tried my hardest to remember. I studied my surroundings. After a few minutes I remembered that everything around me looked familiar, my memory came back. Can you imagine, in the blink of an eye you could lose your memory? This occasion happened more than once to me. Once I got home, I researched this and found out this is called "chemo brain," which is a cognitive impairment or cognitive dysfunction. Signs and symptoms are confusion, difficulty concentrating, fatigue, short-term memory loss, and short attention spans. That was a very scary moment for me. I never told anyone until now.

In addition, I had full strong jet-black hair. Not a weave, but my real hair. I started to lose my hair my it was devastating. One day I was in the bathroom looking in the mirror brushing my hair. I was frightened when I saw clumps of hair falling to the ground. It was like a horror movie—falling hair and fear. It looked like dog hair that had been shed. I began brushing again and as I continued to brush more hair filled my brush and now, I saw bald patches in my head. Even though I knew that this day would come, I still was shocked by the amount of hair loss and the quickness of losing my "covering." Nothing prepared me for this day when it was time for me to put on my wig. I froze. My thoughts were, should I go outside with my bald head? Would people just stare at me? Will they treat me differently just because I look sick? Or would they just not notice? These were the questions I asked myself. In the same manner, one could not fathom the thought of having Stage III Cancer, and chemo treatment. Now I have hair loss, I never thought this would happen to me. It was the feeling worst. I felt ugly, dishonored, and polarized. I felt that my dignity and beauty were stolen. When my daughter walked past and saw all my hair on the floor, I told her that I decided to shave my head, and I did just that. I still had the wigs as a safeguard. I must say that I looked good with my wig on. Tabria called from college, and I told her that I just shaved all my hair off and she asked for a picture, which I sent. Her reaction was, "You rock, Mom. I love you." My response: "Thank you, Sweetie, I love you more."

    The very next day I decided to visit my parents and show off my new look and hang out with my family. My mom also cooked my favorite foods—Mac and Cheese, peach cobbler, collard greens and cornbread. I ate and ate—did not get sick. I felt whole again. I took my mind off everything that was going on around me and enjoyed my family. It was a momentous day. After dinner, we discussed my moving in with my parents due to the stress, high cost, and need for support. Let me tell you, doctor visits, chemo, and medication are extremely expensive. The point—I am going to be broke as I fight against cancer. Not a very good position to be in, especially with a school-aged kid and one in college. It was a tough decision. I had been on my own since high school graduation. I have been independent. Now, I need them. Thank God for parents. I left Lakeland that evening. The next day I was scheduled to see the plastic surgeon. I was not looking forward to seeing him. In my mind, I was not ready for all the changes that were yet to come. There were three procedures the surgeon discussed with me, the first is a (TRAM Flap) of which involved taking the flap of the skin, fat, and all parts of the underlying rectus abdomens muscle and using that to reconstruct my breast. The other options were a mastectomy, the removal of one breast, or a bilateral mastectomy, the removal of both breasts. I was aware of the options before my visit because I did some research. After conversing with my family, I decided to have a bilateral mastectomy to remove both breasts to avoid the future risk of developing breast cancer again. And I was to have reconstruction right after the surgery, which meant the whole procedure was going to last four hours. The surgery was scheduled for June, which was in a few weeks. I had to get things in order because I wasn't sure how this all would unfold. As the weeks flew by, the day finally came! I was preparing myself for surgery, I found myself up early the day of my surgery praying once again. I arrived at the hospital with my daughters, sister, and parents. Not long after I was called in by the nurse to get prepped for my procedure. Everything happened so quickly. The nurse knew I was nervous, so she spoke verses from the Bible to me to and prayed with me.

The anesthesiologist walked in to put me out, and before you knew it, I was in surgery and out in four hours, just as the doctor said. When I woke up from the surgery the first words I said were "Thank you, Lord." I had tears rolling down my cheeks. Then I looked around to see my mother, sister, and aunt Margie at my bedside. I never told my aunt I had cancer, but she was there to support me. I was told that my daughters and everyone else were in the waiting area.

At first, I didn't feel any pain. I was wondering if the surgery went well. My head was pounding with a major headache. I remember looking down at my chest and seeing myself wrapped in white bandages across my chest and back area, with small drains on each side. An assistant of Dr. Lewis came into my room at the time, saw the look on my face and quickly assured me that these drains would remove all the fluid out of my surgical area. Then I looked down and saw that cords were hanging down my legs. My family said the doctor said everything went well during surgery. Tears had never stopped running down my cheeks and I began to praise God for protecting me. My daughters and God kids came in the room and were excited that I made it through and that I was going to be okay. After a while, everyone left me there to rest. As I lay there, I went thinking I didn't want to go through this hardship again. I had made the right decision to remove both breasts and get on with my life.

After a few hours, the doctor came in and stated I was strong, and everything went well during my procedure. He said I had a long road to recovery, and that he had made me an appointment to see him in a week and the doctor stated no driving. I thanked him for everything, and he replied with a smile, "It was the man from above that helped me and helped you." He added that he sent the tissue that was removed from my breast tissue to the lab to check for cancer. The results will be back in a week. I stayed in the hospital for three days, during this time a few of my close friends and family called or came to see me. All that love and support made my day. After I was released from the hospital, I went to stay at my sister Keke's house. It was better for me to stay with her because my doctor's office was ten minutes away. During my release, I was prescribed all these pain medications which I never took, since I didn't believe in taking medication unless it was necessary. I dealt with the pain for weeks because I didn't want to take medication.

Pink Tears

I spent day and night emptying my drain tubes, which were to be in for three weeks. And I had to change my bandages to prevent infections. The surgical drains are called Jackson Pratt drains, which are tubes placed near surgical incisions to remove pus, blood, or other fluids to prevent it from accumulating in the body where the drains were located. They were very uncomfortable and painful, especially when the drains became full. I was so ready to have them removed. I couldn't lift my arms above my head due to the pain. A week later I drove myself to the doctor, even though I was told not to drive. But I wanted to do everything for myself. I asked myself. "How will I get better if someone else is doing my job?" As I was headed to my doctor's, I prayed that everything was well with me, since I was still having a lot of pain.

Once I arrived, the nurse called me back immediately, which made me nervous because I thought I was going to hear more bad news. The last time I was called back I was given horrible news. As I was sitting in the exam room, I remembered the nurse at the hospital giving me a Bible verse to read. I took out my phone and pulled up Matthew 9:20-22. It states that a woman who was diseased with a blood issue for twelve years came behind Jesus and touched the hem of his garment. Jesus turned to her and said, *"Daughter be of good comfort. Thy faith hath made thee whole. And the woman was made whole from that hour."*

Just as I finished reading the doctor walked in. It felt like I had butterflies in my stomach. Dr. Lewis asked how I was feeling, as he went to remove the bandage from around my chest. With my eyes closed I heard the nurse say nice work Doctor. That's when I opened my eyes and noticed two incisions, one going across each breast on each breast. I was amazed at the doctor's work, and while most women probably would be horrified at the sight of their scars, my scars let me know that Jesus had a plan for me. I began to cry and thinking about the fact that it takes someone strong to handle this. This was a struggle for me physically, mentally, and financially. The thought of me wanting to give up was still far from my conscious mind.

After replacing the bandage, the doctor stated that he had my test results from the lab from the tissue they tested from my surgery. I took a deep breath and said a quiet prayer asking God to please let it be good news. Dr. Lewis replied, *"Well everything came back negative, and you are cancer free."* I started shouting thanking God for healing me. Now that Bible verse made a lot of sense to me. While going through my procedure, I was already healed from that moment God's Angel let me know everything was going to be okay. I was told to come back in two weeks to remove the drains. As I left the doctor's office and reached my car, I sat there and all the praise, where just seven months ago I was living my life without a mention for or from God.

As soon as I got home, I broke the news to my daughters, who were filled with joy. They told me they knew I was going to win. *"We are so proud to call you 'Mom.' We love you."* That day was one of the best days of my life. For a moment I forgot I had surgery the way I was jumping around and shouting. The drains I had were so painful, but I won't complain because I had worse days. I was exhausted, so I went to lie down. In the quiet of my room, I started to think about my whole life and all I had experienced.

Pink Tears

A month later I was back at Abby's house and both my drains were removed. The doctor wanted me to come in every three weeks to inject my expanders with saline solution fluid until I was up to my normal breast size for my implants to be placed. The expanders were very uncomfortable, but no one could tell I had my breasts removed. I went back to my oncologist, who also gave me my lab results. She suggested I do radiation daily for twelve weeks. I looked at the doctor like she was stupid, saying, "You just told me I have no sign of cancer and you want me to do radiation to put cancer back in my body?" I refused to do that. She said she recommended it as the normal procedure after surgery. Still, I wasn't going to do it. She stated I still had to complete my 4 remaining chemo treatments which I agreed to do. Now for the first time, I mumbled to myself that God had pulled me through everything so far, and He would not fail me, just like He did with the women with the issue of blood. It was time to put my full trust in my God, and I did.

I had come from a strict childhood to choosing some wrong friends and the wrong man to be with for over a decade, to having two children and hated and loved the man I was living with, and even having police shove a gun in my face. After going through radical surgery that every woman dreads, and I had become the strong, independent woman I am today.

I don't regret anything that went on in my life. I learned who my real friends and family are. Everything happens for a reason, and you must take it and learn from it. There were many times I wanted to give up on life, but I have two beautiful young Daughters who are still looking up to me. Even though I cried many tears and went through many difficult trials and tribulations, I couldn't do anything besides thanking God for chasing after me and never giving up on my salvation. I thank Him for the guidance, protection, and lessons, and for restoring my faith in Him.

Only God can give us the desires of our hearts, and only He can satisfy our wants and needs. I have learned to talk to God daily, even about the smallest of issues. I am so grateful to be alive and writing my story, in hopes of encouraging someone reading my book to get strong and then stay strong. "We are fearfully and wonderfully made," according to the scriptures. That's a powerful statement, and I believe every single word of it. I plan to live my life in service to God because He is the head of my life and all I need to beat Stage III Breast Cancer!!

At this point, I had met God in a dream, vomited up a demon or two, had demons fighting for possession of my body in front of a church full of strangers, and lost all my hair. I had subconsciously developed a fearless attitude towards life. With both breasts being gone, I would be cancer-free and significantly lower my chances of ever having cancer again.

For God hath not given us a spirit of fear, but power and love of a sound mind.

2 Timothy 1:7

CHAPTER 15

Full Circle

I have a great life. Two amazing daughters and the God of everything we know came to visit me personally. The God of millions of creatures knows *me* by name. My attitude towards life is so different from when I was a high school graduate eager to enter the world. I now know that Satan could not wait to send his army after me. I was the perfect target for his plans. God had other plans for me though.

Nothing is more important than sharing my full story with people. I don't do much research on breast cancer and read everyone's stories. Most stories start with the day they found a lump in their breast. My story starts so much further back than that. The moment I chose to "shelve" the Christian beliefs that were instilled in me as a child, was the day I gave Satan a window to let him in. He was trying to get a hold of me back when he had an unbreakable hold on Roy. Satan is a trickster, on Earth to kill, steal, and destroy. Anointed people are his most sought-after people. It's no coincidence that every church family has one problematic child. It took cancer to bring me back to the safe bosom of God.

One of the biggest contributing factors to my healing was changing my mindset. Every time I had a "woe is me" moment or when I had the audacity to question God, I would play *I Won't Complain* by Paul Jones. My mindset was, why complain when I know I am healed? When God visited me in a dream, he didn't come and say, "This is the end for you, Tricia. He said, "get ready for the hardest fight of your life. I controlled my thinking. I did not complain, trusted God, and now I am healed.

Has there been a time when something traumatic happened in your life? Was your faith tested? Well for me, I can answer *yes* to both questions. I love my baby sister, Annlisha. She passed away when she was just a baby. I love my favorite cousin, Walt. He passed away still in his thirties, same as my sweet friend, Anita who died in her twenties. Then I ended up with breast cancer. How do you overcome disappointments, traumatic experiences, hurt, and interruptions that happen in your life that are not planned? We must remember God knows all. He knows your whole life before it happens. Things like this must happen to prepare you for the next season of your life. I learned in this journey your blessing can come from disappointments, traumatic experiences, hurt, and interruptions. This is the time you praise God or your high being in the good or bad, because either way, it is all in God's plan. As the saying goes, "Tell God your plan and tell me how that works out for you." Even though I cried many tears and went through many difficult trials and tribulations I couldn't do anything besides thank God for chasing after me and never giving up on my salvation. I thank Him for the guidance, protection, lessons, and for restoring my faith in Him. Only God can give us the desires of our hearts. I am so grateful to be alive and write my story in hopes of encouraging someone reading my book to remember if you have faith as small as a mustard seed, you can say to this mountain, move from here to there, and it will move. Nothing will be impossible for you. Think about it. Can you imagine being diagnosed with stage 3 cancer, and in 6 months there is no more cancer in your body? Just think about that. I am cancer free because I kept my faith and believed.

These things I have spoken unto you, that in me ye might have peace. In the world ye shall have tribulation: but be of good cheer; I have overcome the world.

John 16:33

Pink Tears

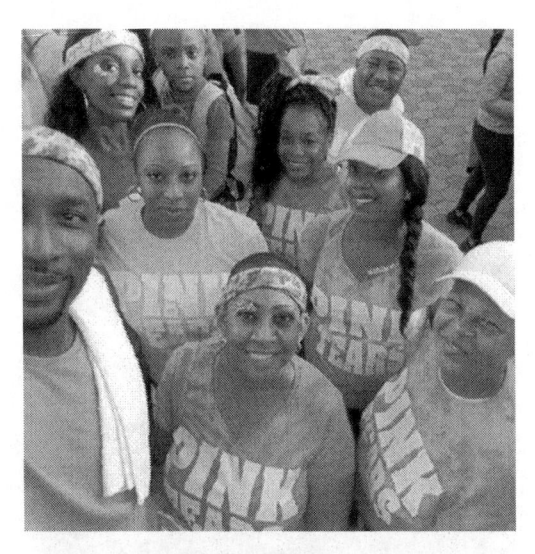

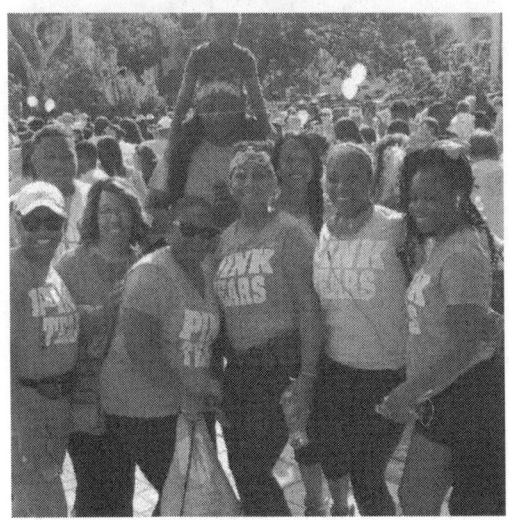

I would like to express my appreciation to my friend Latrencia Johnson, Registered Nurse Practitioner and Colonel in the United States Army. I am forever thankful for you and your family for joining me in my first breast cancer walk in Orlando Florida. Your words of encouragement and love all showed it meant so much to me.
Thank You!

Pink Tears

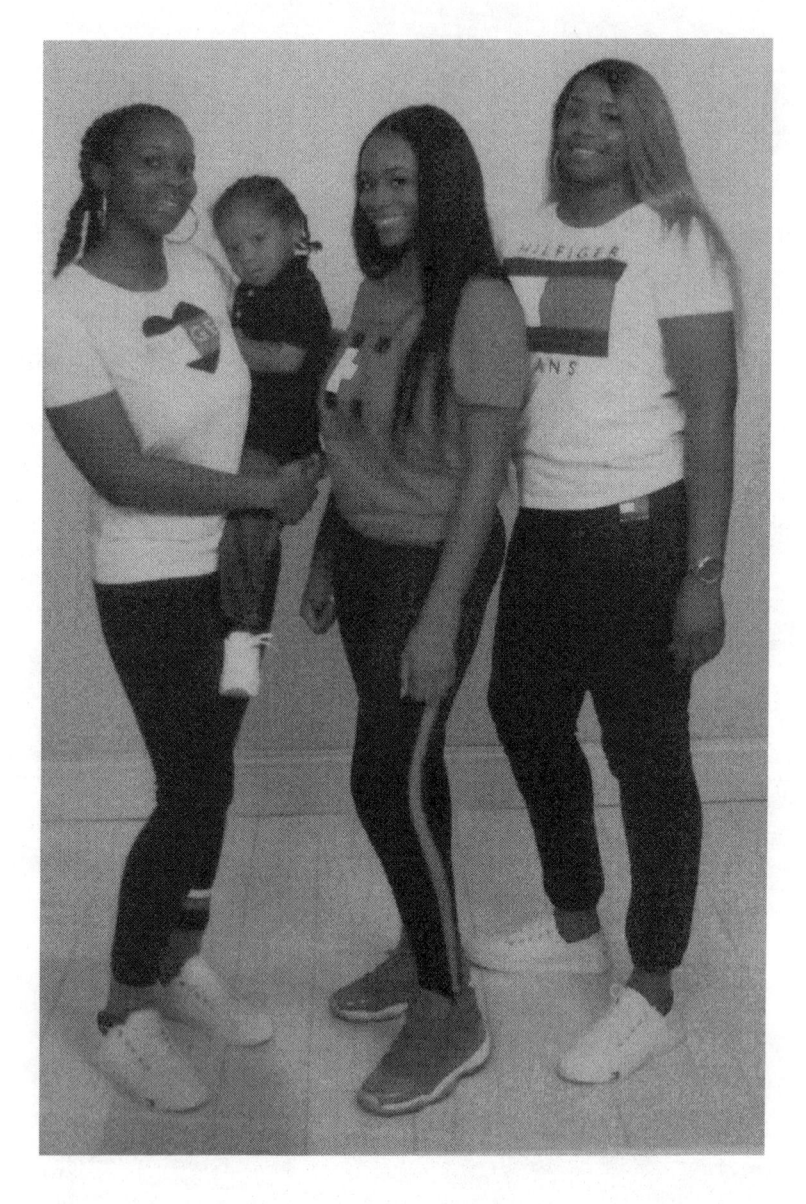

We must keep God First. God kept me for my testimony to help others. In the photo above is My daughters, and Grandson.

Pink Tears

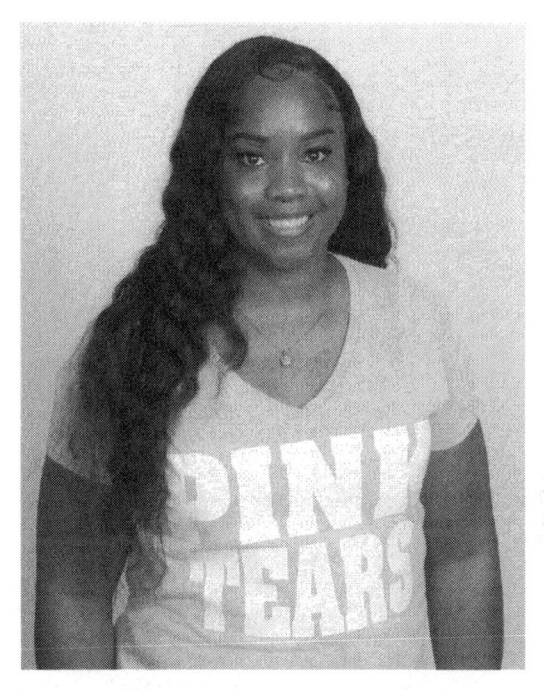

Stop worrying start Believing!
Declare and decree everything in your life.
I learned that life is what you make of it, and we must always fight to win.

Scripture

And Jesus said unto them, Because of your unbelief: for verily I say unto you, if ye have faith as a grain of mustard seed, ye shall say unto this mountain, remove hence to yonder place; and it shall remove; and nothing shall be impossible unto you.
Matthew 17:20-21

Made in the USA
Columbia, SC
10 October 2023